THE ULTIMATE GUIDE TO MEDITATION

ADVANCED MEDITATION TECHNIQUES MADE EASY FOR BUSY PEOPLE, FOR BEGINNERS AND FOR WEIGHT LOSS

By

FLORENCE HIGGINS

Paperback Edition

Copyright © 2016

I0423939

TABLE OF CONTENTS

CONTENTS

FREE GIFT

Are you interested in learning more about living a life which is in YOUR control? Do you want become a successful individual in life?

What I have done for you is created a FREE e-book which you can go ahead and download today. This e-book will get you started on your road to success by revealing

<u>9 Secrets To Master Your Mind</u>!

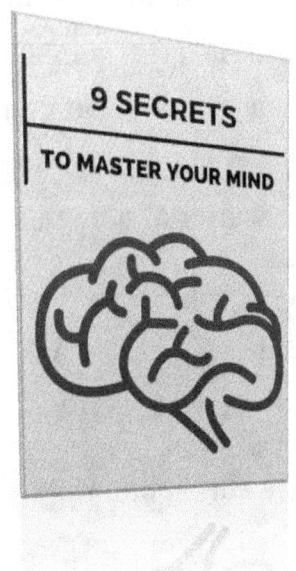

Visit the kindle page for this book to access "The 9 Secrets To Master Your Mind"

See you there!

Florence Higgins

INTRODUCTION

I want to thank you and congratulate you for purchasing the Ultimate Guide To Meditation.

You're going to learn exactly how to meditate, how to use meditation techniques to calm your mind and how to practice meditation daily.

It is important to understand that meditation is not a procedure. Instead, it is a method of life. While meditating, you need to terminate your thought process. It denotes a state of awareness when your mind doesn't have scattered thoughts and ideas.

Genuine meditation can help you focus on your present without worrying about unalterable past and undecided future.

Meditation is basically about training your mind in order to help it cultivate the required skills and strengths it should have to resolve its problems. As there are numerous remedies and solutions for the various diseases of the body, there are several different kinds of meditation for the different issues of the mind.

Meditation is a good way to de-stress and relax. It is also ideal to use in recreating an individual's spiritual and emotional well-being. But for some people, the practice is just another thing to exert their effort in their already jam-packed schedule. This book will address this thinking as meditation aims to bring calmness and serenity from deep within to help you reduce stress instead of heightening it.

As you read this book, you will learn various techniques of meditation, how can it improve your mental health and how it will benefit your overall well-being. Furthermore, this book will teach you the basic and advanced principles of meditating and how you can be successful in this practice.

Thanks again for downloading this book, I hope you enjoy it!

CHAPTER 1- WHAT IS MEDITATION?

Meditation is a state of thoughtless awareness. It is not about effort or doing, rather it is simply a state of awareness. It makes sense that we would think this way because so many things in life validate the use of the mind in getting what we want. We have been raised with the belief that "if you just put your mind to it, you can do anything." There is truth to that, yet the only thing that the mind cannot "do" is meditate.

MEANING ACCORDING TO THE DICTIONARY

From the Latin word Meditari, meditate technically means "to contemplate or be engaged in a reflection". It also means "to reflect or focus one's thought on something". From these definitions, it is clear then that meditation requires focus. But then again, another dictionary such as the Webster's New College Dictionary's ninth edition refers the Latin word mete as to "boundary". In its tenth edition, it mentions that the Latin word mederi means to heal or remedy and also mentions the word medesthai, meaning "to be mindful of".

At first glance, these definitions didn't really help at all. It's a bit confusing and somewhat, misleading but the meaning "to be mindful of" is by far, the closest among them. In practicing meditation, you are also training the mind to stay focused instead of letting it wander over other things. It is all about relaxing the mind, paying focus and attention and achieving a certain goal or purpose. As a beginner, this book will help you learn these basic yet, significant areas of meditation;

Meditation techniques will teach you how to take control of and connect with your mind, but the necessity of that control only pertains to the degree in which it allows you to free yourself from your mind.

Nonetheless, meditation is comprised of various mental training techniques that can help improve the physical and mental health. These techniques range from simple which you can learn by reading this book while other techniques are more complex thus, requiring the guidance of a meditation teacher.

For a more general definition, meditation simply means training your thoughts and has it stay with the present. Present moment offers true peace. Whenever you have thoughts regarding the past, there's a tendency for you to feel sudden sadness, depression and anger about the things that happened where as if you think of the future, this may lead to your anxiety and fears of what might happen. Being focused at the moment will free you from negative emotions, stress and over thinking.

WHY YOU SHOULD MEDITATE

When people are emotionally disturbed, angry, delusional, they may find themselves surrendering to some extremely critical physical ailments. And when they are physically not in their perfect shape, they are likely to find the world a very miserable, dull place. However, this doesn't mean that all our physical problems are caused by extreme emotional states. When you are exposed to elements to which you are or may be allergic, you tend to experience a lot of chances. These changes may include mood swings, hallucinations, depression and even physical effects. Whatever the reason, the physical ailment is usually accompanied by varied unsettling emotions.

Techniques that have been developed and used to avail the healing effects of meditation and relaxation methods have proved to be useful in limiting both the physical issues and extreme emotions that accompany them.

The aim of meditation is to overcome defilement and stray thoughts. Once you're able to control your thoughts successfully, the real state of your mind can become evident. In the absence of negative thoughts, there is no place for hatred, greed, and anger. What's more, the energy that was previously occupied by those damaging thoughts becomes available to you. This ensures your overall physical, emotional, and mental health.

CHAPTER 2- KEY BENEFITS OF MEDITATION

Meditation was barely recognized by Westerners until an Indian yoga teacher named Maharishi Mahesh Yogi introduced Transcendental Meditation (TM) to the United States in 1959. The meditation presented by Maharishi to Americans used a mantra that helped to stimulate relaxation and transcend conventional thinking.

The Beatles, who studied with Maharishi in India, were a big influence on the growing popularity of meditation through the 1960s. With his popularity, Maharishi continued to train more than forty thousand meditation teachers for the next fifty years. The teachers who trained directly under Maharishi then spread out and taught the transcendental meditation technique to more than five million people around the world.

During the last part of the 20th century, other methods of meditation began to gain recognition in the West. One of these new forms of meditation was called insight or mindfulness meditation.

Mindfulness meditation aims to help a person become deeply aware of the present moment in order to be able to completely live through the here and now.

Other forms of meditation utilize visualization and guided imagery through mental pictures to promote relaxation of both mind and body. Currently, over 20 million Americans, which comprise almost 10% of the population, perform regular meditation.

Their purpose for practicing meditation ranges from managing high blood pressure, stress, anxiety, and their overall state of mind in order to live better.

THE AMAZING BENEFITS OF MEDITATION

Nowadays, more and more health practitioners recommend meditation to resolve both mental and physical problems. Even small practices of meditation can cause major neurological improvements. A research published in Psychological Science evaluated the effects of meditation on brain wave activity. It was observed that after seven hours of meditation practice, participants showed an improvement in brain wave activity. Since the improvement was in the left frontal area, it could be easily linked to positive mood changes. Some other benefits of meditation are discussed below. Read on.

IMPROVED MEMORY

Constant meditation practice has a tremendous effect on memory function.

A research conducted by Thomas Jefferson University Hospital involved fifteen senior patients suffering from Alzheimer's disease. While some participants were engaged in twelve minutes of meditation exercises on a daily basis for eight weeks, the remaining participants listened to classical music. On examining the brain scans of both the participant's groups, it was discovered that the people involved in meditation showed increased blood flow in different parts of the brain. Moreover, the same group felt less anxiety, better memory, and had improved memory recall.

PAIN RELIEF

Numerous medical studies support the implementation of meditation to reduce pain. According to a study published in the Journal of

Neuroscience, fifteen adults without any prior experience of meditation joined a research group. They were taught focused attention, a popular meditation style, in four sessions of 20 minutes each. A special kind of magnetic resonance imaging technique was used to scan every participant's brain activity before and after the research. While being scanned, a tiny heat producing system was attached to the body of each participant to trigger a small pain response

STRONGER IMMUNE SYSTEM

A journal named Psychosomatic Medicine published the effects of meditation of the immune system's response. For the purpose of research, analysts administered a vaccine for influenza to a group of people who don't meditate as well as to those who had been engaged in meditation for the period of eight weeks.

PHYSIOLOGICAL ADVANTAGES

The mind-body advantages of meditation are as varied as its practices. Here are a few common advantages that you should know about:

- Quiet meditation stabilizes your heart rate.

- Moderately hypertensive people can control their blood pressure levels using meditation.
- Quicker and better recovery from anxiety and the associated health issues.
- Significant improvement in alpha rhythms. Alpha rhythms are high-amplitude; slow brain waves that are highly correlated with relaxation.
- Meditation improves synchronization of the left and right hemispheres of the brain. This synchronization is correlated with creativity.
- Meditation lowers cholesterol levels.
- It reduces your requirement for oxygen and thus decreases your overall energy consumption.
- Meditation ensures slower, deeper breathing.
- It helps your muscles relax.
- It causes a significant decrease in pain intensity.

PSYCHOLOGICAL ADVANTAGES

Physical or physiological benefits are not the only ones that you can expect to get from meditation. It also offers a plethora of psychological benefits that help you live a peaceful and of course happy life. Here are a few common effects of meditation on your psychology or mental state.

- Meditation can provide you with more peace of mind and happiness.
- It can help you become an empathetic person.
- It can help you become a highly creative individual.
- Self-actualization is another great advantage of meditation.
- It causes a great reduction in both chronic and acute anxiety.
- Meditation complements psychotherapy and many other approaches to treating addiction.

CHAPTER 3- STEP BY STEP INSTRUCTIONS ON HOW TO PERFORM MEDITATION: BEGINNER TECHNIQUES

There are many people who know quite a few meditation exercises, but they don't really practice them. The reason being it is difficult for them to sit still for even a few minutes, let alone ten, fifteen, or twenty minutes.

May be your knees or back start hurting, and you think you might do your body some irreparable damage. Or your body gets itchy in the most uncommon places and you just can't help scratching. Or every odd sound starts catching your attention.

ELEMENTS OF MEDITATION

The different forms of meditation may employ different techniques but they share the following same elements:

FOCUSED ATTENTION

Concentrated attention is the most vital component of meditation. When you focus your attention, you are able to set your mind free from day-to-day distractions that often cause tension and anxiety, and venture into a world of calmness, clarity and peace. What you focus on will vary depending on the type of meditation you are doing.

PEACEFUL BREATHING

To achieve relaxed, deep, even-paced breathing, it is important that you breathe using your diagram. Using your diaphragm is more efficient because it requires minimal action from your shoulders and neck muscles. The objective of slow and deep breathing is to bring more oxygen into your body. This calms you and creates an inner space that is conducive to meditation.

QUIET AND COMFORTABLE SETTING

Advanced practitioners can perform meditation almost anywhere, even if the place is noisy or crowded. As a beginner, it is advisable for you to start practicing meditation in a quiet and comfortable place where you won't be distracted by others.

Before you start your meditation practice, get rid of any distractions. Turn off the television, radio and cell phone before you begin each session.

SITTING UP STRAIGHT

Fortunately, a few well-implemented meditation poses can give your body amazing results and make the experience a lot more enjoyable for you. Regardless of the sitting posture you opt for, you'll be able to enjoy it even more if you have a flexible and strong lower back. After all, you'll get the required support from your body. As you stretch your hips to sit in a cross-legged position, you'll discover that you can sit without putting any additional pressure on your knees.

Once you've selected the postures that work best for you, make sure to practice them carefully and gently. Treat your bod kindly and respectfully. Experience the stretch, but retreat gently in case it gives you any pain. Another important thing to remember is to use a rug or meditation mat between your sensitive body parts and the flooring.

COBRA POSE

Termed for its close resemblance to the elegant serpent, this posture provides your back and spine with an amazing backward stretch. What's more, this pose prevents you from slouching forward. Use only your upper back to begin this stretch, and then slowly spread it down your back.

FOLLOW THESE STEPS TO PRACTICE THIS POSTURE.

- Lie such that your forehead rests on the floor.
- Set your hands below your shoulders. Your fingertips should face forward. Also, the external edge of your hands should be even with those of your shoulders.
- Pull your elbows in such that your arms get in touch with your torso's sides.
- Maintain your feet close to each other. Press your thighs and legs into the floor.
- Move your chest gradually away from the floor. While keeping your neck and head aligned with your spine, lift and extend from the upper back.
- Relax your shoulders. Press the chest forward and upward gently. Open the abdomen while you push your pubic bone into the ground.

- Take smooth and deep breaths.
- Maintain the pose for at least five full breaths.
- Gradually unfold the posture as you breathe out.
- As you once again lie down with the forehead rested on the floor, relax completely.

CAT POSE

Have you ever seen a cat stretching itself after taking a nap? This posture has got its name from there.

This posture not only helps you stretch and support your spine and back for the sitting position, but it also enables you to give your day a fresh start. As soon as you get out of your comfy bed in the morning, sit in the Cat posture for about ten to twenty minutes of meditation practice, and then you're good to go.

FOLLOW THESE STEPS TO PRACTICE THE CAT POSTURE:

- Get on your knees and hands. Keep the spine horizontal. Make sure your thighs and arms are at 90-degree to the floor.

- With every breath you exhale, flex the spine upward like a cat. Stretch your body at the tailbone.
- As the stretch is about to culminate, tuck the chin a little.
- With every breath you inhale, flex the spine downward. Start with the tailbone and lift your head a bit as the stretch ends.
- Continue stretching and breathing in this manner for about ten or twenty minutes.

CRADLE STRETCH

- Helping you open and stretch your hips, this particular posture is all about holding your leg in the arms. Make sure to lift the leg gently and gradually.
- Follow the given steps to practice this posture.
- Sit straight on the floor such that your legs are spread in the front.
- Flex one knee. Let your thigh be rotated to the side. Hold the lower leg in both your arms. Clasp your hands. Use the fold of one elbow to hold the knee and the fold of the other knee to hold your foot.

- Keep the head straight and spine in the extended position. Rock the leg gently from one side to another.
- Maintain the rocking position for at least five breaths. Inhale deep and smooth breaths.
- Slowly put the leg down and repeat the same steps for the other leg.

LOCUST POSE

- This posture resembles a grasshopper when its abdomen is suspended into the air. Since it stretches and supports your lower back, this posture provides you with the strength you need to sit up straight.
- If you're an amateur meditator, start with the half Locust posture and then proceed to the full Locust pose whenever you think your lower back is strong enough. Make slow and smooth progress. Avoid any painful movements.
- Follow these steps to practice this posture.
- Lie down such that your chin rests on the floor. Place your arms at the sides. Keep your palms up.

- With both hands, make a partial fist. Adjust your arms below your body. Set your hands below your pubic bone such that your thumbs touch lightly.

Now you can practice either the full locust or half locust according to your ease.

FULL LOCUST – Inhale and contract the muscles of your buttock a bit. As you breathe out, lift both your legs into the air, but don't bend your knees. Maintain the posture for at least five breaths. Inhale deeply and smoothly into your abdomen. Lower both your legs. Turn the head to any side and calm down.

HALF LOCUST – Inhale and contract the muscles of your buttock a bit. As you breathe out, lift any one leg into the air, but don't bend your knee. Maintain the posture for at least five breaths. Lower the leg and repeat the same steps for the second leg. Repeat multiples times on every side. Turn the head to any side and calm down.

BUTTERFLY POSE

- This posture proves to be a great challenge for athletes as well as a runner. It stretches and gives amazing support to the groin, hip, and inner thigh.
- Follow the given steps to practice this posture.
- Sit straight on the floor such that both your legs are stretched in the front.
- Flex your knees. Bring your feet soles along with the external edges of your feet on the floor.
- Clasp the hands together and then grasp your feet. Pull the heels of your feet in in the direction of your groin. Push the knees in the direction of the floor while you extend your spine.
- Maintain the posture for at least five breaths. Make sure to inhale smooth and deep breaths into the abdomen.
- While breathing out, let go of your feet. Spread your legs in the front and calm down.

LUNGE POSE

- Usually considered a back stretch, this posture supports and stretches your hips. If you don't have much time to try too many postures, just combine the Lunge posture with Cat posture to develop your own mini routine.

- Follow the given steps to practice this posture.

- Get on your knees and hands. Keep the spine horizontal. Make sure your thighs and arms are at 90-degree to the floor.

- Take your left knee a bit forward. While keeping the heel of your left leg close to the right side of your groin, set it on the floor.

- Spread the right leg behind you. Keep it straight. Make sure your knee faces downward.

- Place your pubic bone such that it points toward the floor. Lift the chest forward and upward. Put your weight on the right leg and arms.

- Maintain the posture for at least five breaths.
- Repeat the same steps for the other side.

CHAPTER 4- STEP BY STEP INSTRUCTIONS ON HOW TO PERFORM MEDITATION: ADVANCED TECHNIQUES

TECHNIQUE ONE: FEAR INTO LOVE

Once you find a comfortable position to lie in, preferable crossed legs sitting on a comfy surface. Then what you need to do is take your hands and fold your right hand underneath your left with the palms facing each other. The mysteries behind this is that the left hand is more attached to the heart than the right hand, so that way in a sense you put "love" over everything.

NOTE: This isn't the love you would think of between partners (although it could) but a love for everything, and a love of presenting your gifts to the world. Also that the left hand is connected to the right brain which is dominant in more courageous acts – therefore helping you put yourself out there more for life.

Then the second part is that once you get into this position is you're going to want to close your eyes and only breathe through your mouth. The reason being is that you want to change the pattern of which your used to doing, cause the brain likes patterns. Breathing through the mouth will create confusion for your mind, and it will begin to submit to new things and ideas. Also breathing through the nose stimulates the brain, this meditation is designed to have your brain create less boggled thoughts in order for you to hear your heart instead.

NOTE: This may get uncomfortable after about ten minutes in, that's why I recommend starting out with a short amount of time first. Also to clarify that this is perfectly safe, and an excellent way in order to try something out of the norm. This meditation is great for those who have a problem taking steps forward and want to jump into things and immerse fully into life without the criticism of others bothering them.

TECHNIQUE TWO: NO MIND (GIBBERISH)

Do you tend to chew a lot of gum for some reason, and you don't know why? In my experience after doing this meditation, it helped me release a lot of tension around my neck and jaw especially. The ego is for the most part attached to the face; realize that the ego to a certain degree can also inhibit your bliss in life.

To begin understand this is a cathartic technique, which involves expressive body movements. To start you can either do this in a group or alone – begin with saying nonsense words (gibberish) allow whatever needs to be expressed within just flow out of you. Throw everything out! It doesn't need to make any sense, actually, the less sense the better and just say whatever comes up. Whatever thoughts, sounds, words arise just throw them out. Do this for fifteen minutes.

Then the second part which will also last fifteen minutes is to lie down on your stomach and feel as if you are combing with the earth. As you breathe put extra emphasis on the exhalation as if you were moving one step closer into the earth. This helps recognize the frequencies of which the earth is moving, which in doing so you should take into consideration of moving at this pace in your own life as well.

TECHNIQUE THREE: KUNDALINI MEDITATION

The Kundalini Meditation is usually a step down from the Dynamic, and also has one less stage involved in it as well. There are four stages, and each of which will last you fifteen minutes each.

The first stage is to let your whole body vibrate and shake in which way you'd like. Completely be silly, try to imitate a child's pattern of just shaking. As you do this stage you'll see how the energies begin to accumulate from the feet up through the body. Your eyes may be open or closed as well; also lastly remember to not get stuck in one single pattern or movement be animated and change patterns with how you do this considering the brain likes to get fixed with repeating positions.

The second stage is you want to dance, anyway, you feel, or however you'd like. Let your body move as it wishes; side note as for all these stages as well feel free to turn on any music you'd like preferably something more towards instrumental to not really let the words distract you. (Fewer words in the head, more movement and freedom inside the body.)

Third Stage is to close your eyes and to remain standing or sitting in a still position. Just watch what is happening (Imagine yourself turning your eyes inward and witnessing the bodies expression.) Also, take notice of the outer feelings of your body as well.

The last Stage is to just remain still in whatever position you chose while keeping your eyes closed, and just remain still. By being active in the beginning stages you'll recognize how much easier it is by now to ease the thoughts inside your head, and let go of them.

TECHNIQUE FOUR: DYNAMIC MEDITATION

Before going into this meditation I would like to warn, and state that this is not for beginners necessarily. Please be advised that this is not an ordinary meditation, and should be done with caution. The reason being is that if done properly a significant change will be done within the body after doing this successfully. You'll notice a change within your body and perhaps a slight temporary discomfort in your stomach after doing this. This is normal and natural because it releases the tensions that're held within your body, and is now creating an opportunity for your body to finally in a sense "open up", and not be closed off.

Let's begin: this meditation will have five stages each of them being ten minutes. Feel free though as with any meditation to work your way up to this amount of time. Also, I invite you to try and pick some sort of music that you could have stay repeated throughout this process. You can also do this with people, or alone too.

The first stage is chaotic breathing; it's a form of charging the body. You'll begin by breathing only through your nose violently in and out as fast and chaotic as possible while animating your body. This needs to happen in order to charge the body, and bring the emotions to the surface.

NOTE: In my experience I have done this, and have liked it by I have also tried an exercise called "The Bow" in order to charge the body better, and invite you to look this up as well and try it for yourself.

The second stage will be a catharsis, which is a purging of emotions. Once you have built up a charge inside the body this is the part where you want to let it all out. Express everything you have held inside the body without your head needing to be involved. Whatever emotions come to the surface don't judge them; they could be tears, laughter, anger, yelling, etc.

 The third stage is the grounding stage in order for you to make your energy centered. In this stage, you want to remain standing put your hands over your head as high as you can, and jump in the air repeatedly, and land flat footed. With every time you hit the ground you should repeat a deep sounding "Hoo", the word allows breaking up tension in order for energy to reach down into the sex center. Do this until you spend yourself (or ten minutes.)

 Fourth stage which I will also invite you to do this stage, and the next for even up to fifteen minutes each (mainly because these aren't exhausting, but more of celebrating.) Immediately after you get done with the third stage you want to just stop freeze, and if you'd like just to lay on the ground. Do not move a muscle, and do not do anything just witness the energies pulsing throughout your body. If a proper state has been reached up until this stage, it's a real enlightening feeling that can't really be explained.

The last stage is rejoicing after the fourth stage feels free to get up and just begin dancing soothingly. Start by swaying your body and let it drift, and dance with the "currents of life". You need not do much here, just remember that you are celebrating at this point.

CHAPTER 5- HOW TO MEDITATE AS A BUSY PERSON

At the present time, busy people find it hard to get relaxed. Though lots of activities like yoga are there which can help them in getting relax, the deficiency of time does not allow them to do such activities. Moreover, people use antidepressant tablets to get relaxed. Though antidepressants give a sense of relaxation, they can be highly hazardous afterwards. In such cases, meditation can be highly helpful as it helps in augmentation of emotional, spiritual and material levels. Meditation has been carried out since long and is highly fruitful of busy people. Meditation helps in lessening the stress and thus acts as an antidepressant. Moreover, those who carry out meditation with a proper routine have strong emotional health and get their stress reduced.

MEDITATION- BRIEFLY DEFINED

Meditation is a procedure of mental exercises the augments the activities of brain and heart. The brain thinks in a better way and the heart results in better emotions.

WORKING OF MEDITATION

The process of meditation works with our consciousness. Our brain is actually having four parts. Each part works separately. The separate working results in stress and pain. When the whole brain starts working altogether, the stress and the obstacles in your success eliminates. You are more focused and motivated to your goal and get your job done successfully. During Meditation, you make your all neurons work together. The complex development of brain results in deep thinking and brain works properly.

SHORT PERIOD MEDITATIONS

Meditation is not a time taking exercise; you can do it for minutes to get relaxed mentally and physically. If you do meditation for ten minutes regularly, you will get great benefits emotionally and spiritually. Moreover, if you spend few minutes daily in meditation you will get your skills developed and improved. With the passage of time your meditation state becomes easy to achieve. The best time for meditation is early morning. The fresh air and environment in the morning can greatly help in short term meditation. Moreover, in the morning, your mind is completely at ease and the home environment allows you to meditate. You just have to leave your bed 30 minutes earlier than the others to get the state of meditation. This will even help in the homes where kids do not allow you to meditate. Once you achieve success in doing meditation, it will be much easier next time.

YOU CAN MEDITATE EVERYWHERE

It is difficult to focus on something however you can meditate even on the move. It generally happens that people cannot find time to meditate early in the morning and rush to their offices to start working. For such people, a meditation on the move can be highly helpful. You can meditate everywhere even at your work desk. You can also meditate at a public place and can get rid of the noise of the public as well. You can use earplugs at public places to cut out from the public noise for few minutes.

STEPS INVOLVED IN SHORT TERM MEDITATION

Personalization: If you are a busy person and always remain under your boss, you can use the personalization technique of meditation. The best thing that you can do is the usage of personal pronouns. Do not copy the words spoken by your boss, do command or repeat them in your own words. Try to give new phrases to the instructions to give. Meaningful wording can be highly helpful in this regard. Using your own words, helps you improve your emotional health. Moreover, you get your spirits improved.

Localization: It is common that when you struck among several issues, your attention diverts every moment. You cannot concentrate on one thing easily. However, you can meditate if you localize yourself. You have to sum up you all energies and focus on the major issue that you currently face. Make a list of issues and list them with priorities. Ponder over the problem that is listed at the top. This way, you can think clearly about the specific problem you face and get the solution early.

Memorization: Memorization greatly helps in getting the state of meditation. You just need to sum up the ideas in your mind and recall them at the time you need them. For some, the memorization is quite difficult. However, they do it differently. They like to writer whatever they want to be recalled. Doing so greatly helps in recalling something. Better memorization involves high-lightening the written idea. You can use pink, yellow or sky blue highlighter to give levels to the ideas. The pink idea is, of course, stands at the top. The high-lightening increases the chances of memorization three folds.

Verbalization: It is good to repeat the things you want to memorize. Repetition is considered key to success. If you use your verbal action to repeat the activities you want to do, you will get your mind sharpen. Your will power energizes to get the state you want to be at. Murmuring can be highly helpful but it must be clear to you.

Visualization: Whatever you visualize, you get it. You mind and heart together visualizes the ideas. The idea that you visualize hard to practice will surely be a hard task for you. However, if you consider something a piece of cake, you get the job done in few minutes without getting in any kind of hassle. You can practice by making images in your mind. The better the image the better will be the result.

Actualization: Whatever you do, values you. The actualization of the idea can be highly helpful successful for you. In case, you have done all the steps: personalization, localization, memorization, verbalization and visualization, but not the actualization your whole meditation practice goes spoiled. Practice whatever you think or verbalize.

However, you have to understand the seven Ps formula of meditation if you remain busy throughout the day.

Purpose: you must have purpose for meditation

Prospect: The prospect gives you direction to success

Place: a specific place is a must for meditation

Period: you must set a specific period of meditation

Preliminaries: Get relaxed and remove all that tightens you

Position: The body posture helps in getting better meditation state

Practice: Practice is the only step that worth all. If you don't practice all the Ps go wrong.

CHAPTER 6- HOW TO LOSE WEIGHT USING MEDITATION

A lot of people attest to the effectiveness of meditation as an aid in weight loss. There are two ways on how meditation can help people lose weight and they are the following:

IT HELPS BUILD AND RESTORE MOTIVATION

Lack of focus and motivation is among the reasons people fail in their diet. Focus is exactly what meditation gives you; so people who meditate have higher chances at making a particular weight loss plan work.

Also, people who meditate practice more discipline than those who don't, so the intense discipline that dieting entails won't be a shock to their system. As a result, people who meditate are less likely to quit too soon.

IT HELPS PEOPLE EAT LESS BY LIVING AND SAVORING EVERY MOMENT

Among the things that meditation teaches you are the focus and living in the moment. These are exactly your weapons in fighting food cravings and overeating.

People who meditate eat slower because they savor each bite. When you savor each and every inch of your food, you give your taste buds absolute satisfaction and nothing to crave for afterwards.

People often overeat because their brain tells them they are still hungry when in fact they are already full. Science has proven that signals which carry the message "you're already full" may take some time to get to the brain, so you have to give it a chance by eating slowly. These are habits formed by meditation and are very effective in curbing weight gain.

HOW MEDITATION HELPS YOU LOSE WEIGHT

First, start with a meditation where you think about your eating habits. Slip on your headphones, put on your favorite **harmonics** track, relax, and think about when you tend to overeat; what factors trigger your overeating; which foods you reach for without even thinking about it...

Stress, depression and boredom are all emotions that push people to overeat. Eating is a simple task that only requires a one-track mindset. It's so easy to eat! Unfortunately, you can end up taking in an entire day's worth of calories, or more, in one sitting. Meditation can help you control these behaviors through carefully practiced self-discipline and deeper emotional connections with yourself.

In order to experience effective weight loss that lasts, you have to make real and permanent changes in your habits. Essentially, you will replace your negative overeating habits with positive habits that make you feel good both physically and emotionally.

Habits are more than a physical activity. There is the psychological motivation behind them. You repeat a behavior and turn it into a habit so that you can gain pleasure, whether physical or emotional, from it. Meditation can help you reprogram yourself so that you experience just as much pleasure from a lifestyle of healthy eating as you did from eating a whole bag of cookies.

Willpower by itself is not enough to break a habit. In fact, it can make it feel harder to break habits. Willpower implies that you are depriving yourself of something you want. It would be more prudent to use meditation to teach yourself to want the things you need... to replace a desire for unhealthy food with a 'replacement habit' that has your best interests in mind – such as having a tall glass of water before you eat (often, thirst is mistaken for hunger pangs!) or getting in the habit of cutting your portions in half.

Maintaining weight loss requires a lifestyle change that must take hold in the mind FIRST before you can implement it successfully. Meditation can help root it.

Change can be scary, but if what you're currently doing isn't working, then change is necessary. Meditation provides a gentler way to ease yourself into new thoughts you may have been fighting against before.

Meditation helps increase your own self-**awareness** and makes you less likely to succumb to emotional eating.

Meditation is a mental and physical discipline. It helps you to de-stress on a daily basis so you avoid uncontrolled emotional eating. Meditation teaches you self-mastery so you can say no to indulgences. You can also use the time that you spend on meditating introspectively. Meditation promotes a healthy mind. Practice visualizing yourself at your ideal weight and level of fitness. You can then motivate yourself to take better care of your body.

~ THE END ~

THANK YOU AGAIN FOR DOWNLOADING THIS BOOK!

I hope this book was able to help you to get comfortable meditating and begin meditating on a regular basis. I hope this book gave you all the necessary information you needed to understand meditation better and apply it to your life in order to reduce stress and anxiety and achieve unending success

If you enjoyed this book, then I'd like to ask you for a favor, would you be kind enough to leave a review for this book on Amazon? It'd be greatly appreciated!

Click here to leave a review for this book on Amazon!
Thank you and good luck!